Preventing Bladder Infections

A New Understanding

Jeffrey Pollen, MD

Published in 2019

Copyright 2019 by Jeffrey Pollen, MD

Medical Book Publications, Rockville, Maryland, USA – 1-240-751-2175

ISBN-13: 978-0692191569 (Medical Book Publishers)

Dedication

This book is dedicated to my brilliant teachers and trusting patients. Together you have imbued me with a deeper understanding of medicine in general and urology in particular. I have learned from you all.

Disclaimer

This book, *Preventing Bladder Infections—A New Understanding*, is informational only. No medical or treatment recommendations are implied. Changes to your medical care can only be given by a licensed professional. No book is a substitute for personal medical attention.

The information in this book should not be construed as personal medical advice. No action should be taken based solely on the contents of this book. Readers should consult appropriate health professionals on matters relating to their health or well-being. This book is not meant to be used to diagnose or treat any medical condition. For a diagnosis or treatment of any medical problem, consult your physician.

The content of this book is not intended to create any physician-patient relationship or replace any in-person medical consultation or examination. Always seek the advice of a trained health professional with questions you may have regarding your medical condition or treatment. Never disregard professional medical advice or delay seeking medical treatment due to information obtained in this book. The content of this book is not intended to diagnose, treat, or cure; nor is it intended to replace proper medical care.

The publisher and author are not responsible for specific health needs that may require medical supervision and are not liable for any damages or negative consequences of any treatment, action, application, or preparation to any person reading or following the information in this book.

This book and its content are the product of UroMedicOne LLC. The views and comments expressed in this book are not endorsed or supported by any school, university, or healthcare system. The views expressed in this book are not the views of the United States Department of Veterans Affairs or the United States Federal Government.

Contents

Introduction 1

Chapter 1: Anatomy and Function of the Urinary Tract 7

Chapter 2: Urinary Tract Infections (UTI) 11

Chapter 3: Causes of Urinary Tract Infections 15

Chapter 4: Ascending Urinary Tract Infections 21

Chapter 5: Urinary Tract Infection Is The Second Most
Common Infection 27

Chapter 6: Diagnosis of a UTI 29

Chapter 7: Treatment of a Bladder Infection 33

Chapter 8: Self-Diagnosis and Self-Treatment of a UTI 39

Chapter 9: Risk Factors for a UTI 41

Chapter 10: Prevention of a UTI 45

Chapter 11: Sex and Bladder Infections 57

Chapter 12: Urinary Tract Infection in Adult Males 61

Chapter 13: Preventing Urinary Tract Infection in Females – Review 65

Chapter 14: Key Messages 67

Glossary of Terms 69

About this Book 75

Biography of Author 77

Introduction

LADDER INFECTIONS ARE known by different names, including urinary tract infection, or UTI, and acute bacterial cystitis. Women with recurrent bladder infections are commonly referred to a urologist for evaluation. Over many years of practice as a urologist, I detected a very common pattern among women who were struggling with recurrent bladder infections. Nearly all of these women were proud to announce that they were drinking a lot of water to "flush out" their urinary systems. In fact, many of them attended the appointments carrying a plastic water bottle from which they gulped heartily. Because of their high intake of liquid, these women were happy to report that they urinated very frequently. They were also scrupulous with their feminine hygiene and made a point to urinate and wash their genital area immediately after intercourse. Interestingly, most of these women also shared a background of constipation.

Since intercourse has been identified as the leading cause of urinary tract infections, traditional conventional recommendations relating to sex have included:

1. drinking a glass of water and washing the genital area before sex; and

2. urinating without delay after intercourse, drinking a glass of water, and washing the genital area.

'Preventing Bladder Infections' will show how these ritual behaviors may actually promote, rather than prevent, urinary tract infections.

Urinary tract infections are caused by bacteria that live in the stool within the rectum and develop in three stages:

1. stool from the rectum is transferred to the genital area,

2. bacteria from the fecal material contaminate the end of the urethra, and

3. bacteria are most likely to ascend into the bladder during urination, when the urethra is *open*.

The urethra is the channel through which urine exits from the bladder. While the bladder is filling up with urine, the urethra is tightly closed. During urination the urethra is wide open. Therefore washing and cleaning the genital area after urination and before intercourse can increase the risk of contamination. Similarly, urinating immediately after intercourse may allow bacteria to enter the bladder as the urethra is open again.

If the conventional recommendations to prevent urinary tract infection were effective, one would expect the incidence of UTI to have declined. The incidence of urinary tract infection, however, has not changed! The need to urinate is a normal and natural event. Furthermore, the possibility of occasional contamination of the urethra is inevitable. For these reasons, we cannot prevent urinary tract infections completely. By learning techniques to avoid contamination and reduce the frequency of urination, however, we can go a long way towards minimizing recurrent urinary tract infections.

This book was written with the hope that women who suffer from recurrent urinary tract infections will understand how UTIs develop, learn how to protect themselves from infections, and not be intimidated by their bladders.

Who Will This Book Help?

This book is addressed to those women who have been told that they have a normal urinary tract, who drink plenty of water and cranberry juice, are meticulous with genital hygiene yet experience three or more infections each year. The information in this book will explain how their behavior is contributing directly to their frequently developing UTIs.

Who Else Will Benefit From This Book?

This book will also help caregivers who have a patient that frequently develops new bladder infections, even though the patient follows all the conventional advice for prevention.

Professionals who are dedicated to diagnosing and treating recurrent UTIs may also gain new insight concerning the production and prevention of bladder infections.

How is This Book Different?

Current medical literature suggests that bacteria enter the bladder through the act of intercourse. There is a strong perception that bacteria are massaged into the bladder during the sex act. However, *the urethra is closed* during sexual activity and, therefore, impenetrable to bacteria from the outside. If sexual activity was the main cause of bladder infections, we would see a worldwide pandemic of urinary tract infections related to intercourse. Yet this is not the case and UTIs rarely make headline news.

Novel Wisdom From This Book

Sex is unlikely to cause a UTI. But the actions or behaviors that are currently promoted *surrounding* the sex act purporting to prevent such infections may instead contribute to the development of bladder infections.

What Does This Book Address?

This book addresses the most common form of UTIs, acute bacterial cystitis, that occur in adult women who are known to have normal kidneys and bladder. There is a focus on women who have repeated attacks of UTIs but this book does not address special cases such as UTIs in infants, children, and pregnant women. Those situations require immediate, special, and dedicated care.

This book does not address complex urinary infections that occur in people with functional or structural abnormalities of the urinary tract. Infections that develop in a urinary tract that is obstructed or contains stones require a specialist and individualized special medical care. Occasionally men develop acute cystitis, and this will be mentioned briefly in a later section.

SUMMARY

Conventional Recommendations to Prevent UTIs:

1. Sex causes UTIs, so drink water before and after sex so you will void frequently and therefore flush bacteria from the bladder.

2. Wash genital area before and after sex and urinate immediately after sex.

3. Drink large quantities of liquids, including cranberry juice.

4. Wear cotton underwear and avoid tight-fitting garments.

5. Take showers, not baths.

New Understandings of UTIs:

1. Sex is not likely to cause UTIs; instead, the rituals surrounding sex may cause the problem.

2. Frequent urination does not flush bacteria out of the bladder because there are normally no bacteria in the bladder to flush out.

3. Bladder infections are caused by bacteria that live in the stool and contaminate the genital area.

4. Bacteria enter the bladder during urination, when the urethra is open. Urination enables bacteria from fecal matter in the genital area to be washed upstream into the bladder.

5. Between urinations, the urethra is like a closed door that protects the bladder from infection. Drinking a lot of water causes frequent urination, opening the door to the bladder each time, thus repeatedly exposing the bladder to infection.

6. Urinating after sexual intercourse can encourage bladder infections by inviting bacteria lingering in the genital area to enter the open urethra.

7. Preventing constipation and cleaning the anal area meticulously after bowel movements can help protect against bladder infections.

CHAPTER 1:
Anatomy and Function
of the Urinary Tract

Anatomy of the Urinary Tract

THE URINARY TRACT in both males and females contains kidneys which are a pair of bean-shaped organs located in the back of the upper abdomen, below the diaphragm. The kidneys are partially protected by the lower rib cage. The renal pelvis functions as a funnel with skinny branches that extend upwards from the ureter and attach to each kidney. These branches, called calyces, collect the urine that is produced by the kidneys (see Figure 1).

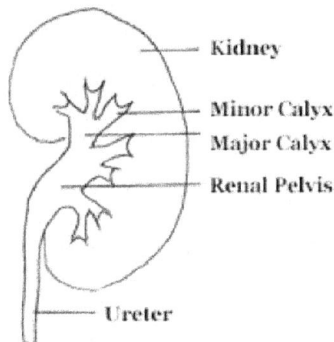

Figure 1: Anatomy of a kidney.

The narrow end of the renal pelvis joins a long thin tube called the ureter. The ureter transports urine from the kidneys to the bladder (see Figure 2).

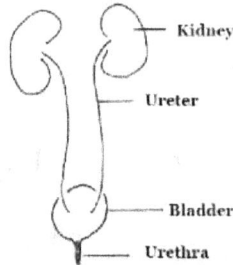

Figure 2: The urinary system in females.

Urine from both kidneys is collected and stored in the urinary bladder. When the bladder is full, there is an urge to urinate. At the time of urination, the bladder empties its contents and urine leaves the body through the open urethra in a urinary stream. At the end of normal urination, the bladder should be virtually empty, leaving little or no urine behind. In females, the urethra opens inside the vestibule in front of the vagina. The vestibule is normally concealed by the inner folds of the genitalia, called the labia minora (see Figure 3).

THE URETHRA IS THE KEY TO UNDERSTANDING THE DEVELOPMENT OF ASCENDING URINARY INFECTIONS.

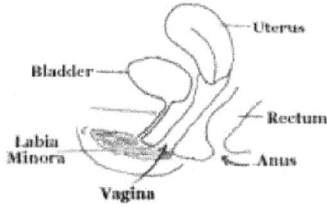

Figure 3: Female pelvic organs.
The shaded area is the vestibule.

In males the urethra opens at the end of the penis (see Figure 4).

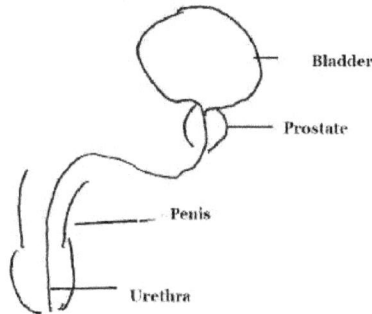

Figure 4: The male bladder and urethra.

Function of the Kidneys

The kidneys produce urine. Urine contains toxic waste products that build up naturally in the body as a result of metabolism. The body must eliminate these toxins in order to survive. Taking in too much water can be just as harmful to the body as toxic waste products; therefore the kidneys remove excess drinking water from the body in addition to removing toxic waste. The kidneys maintain a tight balance on how much water the body contains; not too much and not too little.

The toxins that the kidneys remove are dissolved in the urine. Drinking more water does not remove more toxins from the body. The same measure of toxins is removed, whether it is dissolved in a small or large volume of urine. If there is too much water circulating in the bloodstream, the toxins are diluted and removed in a larger volume of urine. If there is too little water circulating in the bloodstream, the toxins are concentrated and eliminated in a smaller volume of urine. As long as the kidneys are healthy and doing their job, the toxins are excreted. At the end of the day, the same fixed quantity of toxins is eliminated irrespective of the amount of water consumed.

CHAPTER 2:
Urinary Tract Infections (UTI)

Who Gets Urinary Tract Infections?

UTIs CAN AFFECT any age group, from newborns to the elderly. Most infections affect young females of reproductive age. UTIs are ten times more common in females than males. Most women can expect to experience at least one bladder infection in their lifetimes. About 50 percent of women experience a second UTI. About 20 percent of women who have had three or more infections are likely to experience the recurrent infections that this book addresses. These unfortunate individuals live in constant fear and anxiety of a repeat infection, even though they may be meticulous in the preventative measures they have been conventionally taught.

Classification of Urinary Tract Infections

A urinary tract infection is an infection in any part of the urinary tract. Urinary tract infections most commonly attack the kidney, ureter, or bladder:

- *Pyelonephritis* is a serious bacterial infection that attacks the kidney and presents with a high fever, shaking chills, and flank pain. A woman with pyelonephritis is very sick and may need to be admitted to a hospital for intravenous antibiotics. Pyelonephritis is an upper urinary tract infection.

- *Pyelitis* is a somewhat lesser UTI. It is limited to the collecting system of the kidney and is associated with a mild fever, a possible shaking chill and less severe flank pain. Pyelitis, which is probably more common than is mentioned in modern textbooks, can often accompany a bladder infection. Pyelitis is a middle urinary tract infection.

- *Acute Cystitis* is an infection that involves the bladder. It is classified as a lower urinary tract infection.

Both types of upper urinary tract infections—pyelitis and pyelo-nephritis—are extensions of a lower UTI or bladder infection. These upper tract infections can be prevented by prompt attention to and treatment of infections in the bladder, or lower urinary tract. If a bladder infection remains untreated, it can ascend and become a middle tract or upper tract infection.

> ACUTE CYSTITIS IS AN INFECTION THAT INVOLVES THE BLADDER. IT IS CLASSIFIED AS A LOWER URINARY TRACT INFECTION.

Acute Bacterial Cystitis

Infections of the urinary tract may be caused by a wide variety of organisms, including parasites, fungi, or viruses. By far though, the most common cause of UTIs is a bacterial infection. This book focuses on bacterial infections that concentrate in the lower urinary tract. The most common UTI is acute bacterial cystitis, usually referred to as a bladder infection. It is also called a "simple" urinary tract infection because it usually responds promptly to a short course of antibiotic treatment. Acute cystitis develops when bacteria enter the bladder and set up an acute inflammation. Occasionally, an infection that started in the bladder travels up the urinary tract and infects a kidney. An infection of the kidney requires more intense antibiotic treatment.

Symptoms of Urinary Tract Infections

Acute cystitis may cause burning during urination and/or increased frequency of urination. The symptoms may be mild and self-limiting, sometimes resolving without antibiotic treatment. Most commonly, cystitis is an acute infection that causes the following symptoms:

❑ An attack appearing out of the blue

❑ A sudden onset of urgency to urinate

❑ Frequency of urination

❑ Intense discomfort, pain, or burning on urination

❑ Cloudy urine with unpleasant odor

❑ With or without blood in the urine

❑ Sometimes with pain in the lower abdomen

Table 1: Symptoms of UTI

The urine can appear pinkish in color due to the presence of small amounts of blood in the urine. Once in a while, an alarming amount of blood becomes visible in the urine. This is known as *gross hematuria*. While blood in the urine can be a sign of something more sinister happening in the urinary tract, by far the most common cause of blood in the urine is a UTI. The blood usually signifies a severe inflammation of the bladder called *hemorrhagic cystitis*.

Unlike a kidney infection that exhibits a high fever and chills, acute cystitis is not usually accompanied by a high fever. Nonetheless, the discomfort is intense, and most women want relief and treatment immediately. They do not want to wait until the next day for a doctor's appointment.

If UTIs Go Untreated

Fortunately, nature has been good to us. Most UTIs will resolve themselves over time. However, others may ascend to the kidneys and cause pyelonephritis; a kidney infection with far more serious problems. The escalation of a bladder infection to an infection of the kidney pelvis or the kidney itself, can occur in patients who drink lots of water in an attempt to "flush out" the initial infection—a strategy that may fail. Also, if the caregiver's initial choice of antibiotic was ineffective or there was a delay in treating the bacterial cystitis, the infection may take advantage of the situation and ascend to the kidneys.

> PROMPT AND EFFECTIVE TREATMENT
> OF ACUTE CYSTITIS IS THE BEST
> PROTECTION AGAINST DEVELOPING A
> KIDNEY INFECTION.

Chills, Nausea, Fever, Shaking, Back Pain

It is not uncommon for cystitis to be accompanied by a low-grade fever, a chill and mild back pain. These symptoms indicate the infection has ascended to the ureter and renal pelvis to cause pyelitis. A high fever, shaking, chills, and back pain may signal a kidney infection called pyelonephritis. This condition requires immediate and effective treatment. Drinking large amounts of water can lead to a large amount of urine in the ureter which can link the urine in the bladder to the urine in the kidneys. If that happens, a bladder infection can turn into a serious kidney infection.

CHAPTER 3:
Causes of Urinary Tract Infections

Predisposing Factors to UTIs

MOST ARTICLES ON urinary infections deliver a common list of predisposing factors to urinary infections. Here are the ones most frequently mentioned:

- the female sex
- history of previous bladder infections from a young age
- drinking too little liquid
- voiding infrequently

Risk factors that are often listed include:

- wiping the backside by reaching from the front between the legs
- diarrhea
- urinary incontinence
- pregnancy
- congenital structural abnormalities

- kidney stones

- obstructions to the urinary tract

- diabetes

- immune deficiency diseases

Risk factors that are seldom mentioned concern conditions around the anal area:

- Prolapse (slipping down) of the rectum is a condition most commonly associated with prolapsing hemorrhoids. Such a condition is frequently associated with fecal contamination which, in turn, is a risk factor for UTIs.

- Constipation is a risk factor for UTIs for two reasons. One: hard stools found in the anal area causes difficulty with hygiene. Two: severe constipation leads to overflow diarrhea. The stool above the constipation undergoes fermentation and liquefaction. The liquid stool escapes around the hard stool to cause diarrhea, a risk factor for contamination and ascending urinary infections. Treating this condition involves treating the constipation which, in turn, controls the diarrhea. Mistakenly treating the diarrhea with medications that reduce diarrhea may aggravate the situation instead of improving it. The cycle of constipation, diarrhea, and urinary tract infections plays out frequently in the elderly sedentary population, most notably in extended-care facilities.

- Some women are prone to contamination in the anal area because of a narrow perineum (the area between the vulva and the anus). In such cases, the periurethral area is so close to the rectum that fecal contamination becomes all too common. A person may be born with a narrow perineum, or it may become narrow after childbirth. The best protection from fecal spillover contaminating the urethral area is meticulous hygiene around the anal area.

What Causes Urinary Tract Infections?

Normally, the urinary tract is sterile: *Urine in the kidneys and bladder contains no germs at all.* Most UTIs are caused by bacteria. The bacterium that causes most cases of UTIs is *Escherichia coli*, commonly referred to as *E. coli*. This bacterium accounts for 80 to 95 percent of all UTIs. By far, the majority of UTIs are auto-infections. This means the bacteria that cause the infection are derived from one's self, from inside the person's own body. Most UTIs are not sexually transmitted diseases.

The main reservoir for *E. coli* is within the large intestine. *E. coli* live happily in the stool in the interior of the large intestine, which is comprised of the colon and the rectum. When at home in the large intestine, *E. coli* are mostly harmless. They may actually help protect us from certain intestinal diseases. *E. coli* may also produce a variety of vitamins for our benefit.

So long as *E. coli* remain in the stool, there is no problem. Complications arise when stool containing *E. coli* contaminates the area around the opening of the urethra, also called the periurethral area. *E. coli* contaminating the periurethral area is a potential cause of UTIs. The *E. coli* that causes urinary infections are referred to as *uropathogens*.

> A URINARY INFECTION IS CAUSED BY E. COLI THAT LIVE IN THE STOOL. STOOL CONTAMINATES THE OPENING OF THE URETHRA. E. COLI THAT ASCEND INTO THE BLADDER THROUGH THE URETHRA MAY ESTABLISH AN INFECTION IN THE URINARY TRACT.

The Vestibule and the Periurethral Area

The vestibule is the area of the internal genitalia that is located within the labia minora. The vestibule is a common area shared by the opening of the vagina and the opening of the urethra. The shaded area in the figure below is the vestibule (see Figure 5).

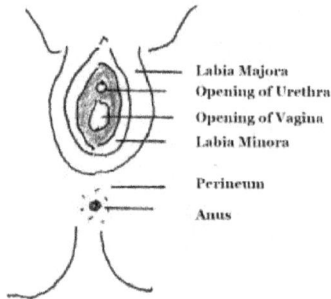

Figure 5: The anus, perineum, female
genitalia, and vestibule.

The urethra opens in the vestibule immediately in front of the vagina. The periurethral area includes the vestibule, the opening of the vagina, the opening of the urethra, as well as a short segment of the lowermost segment of the urethra. The female urethra is about four cm long. The lower one cm segment of the urethra is included in the definition of the periurethral area (see Figure 6).

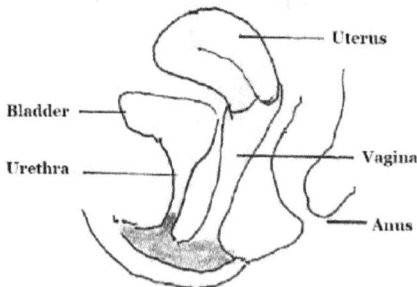

Figure 6: Female pelvic organs.
The shaded area is the periurethral area,
which includes the vestibule
and the lower end of the urethra.

Contamination of the Periurethral Area

How Does Stool Get to the Periurethral Area?

Stool may contaminate the periurethral area by spillage across the perineum. Stool splashing into a toilet bowl may splatter contaminated water onto the genital area. Fecal material may soil the underwear or sanitary pads and, consequently, transfer to the genital and urethral areas.

It is well-known that wiping after a bowel movement by reaching from the front (from between the legs) to the back can transfer stool from the anal area to the genital area. Wiping by reaching from the back is a much healthier option (see Figure 7).

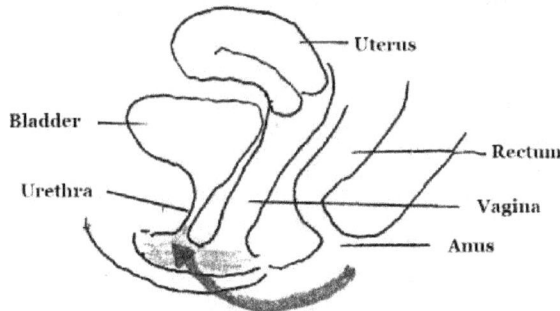

Figure 7: Pathway of stool from the anus to the periurethral area. Wiping the rear end by reaching from the front between the legs can transfer stool from the anal area to the periurethral area.

Persistent colonization of the genital area is not very common. It can be a problem for women who insert cervical caps or use diaphragms for contraception. Women who wear vaginal pessaries for control of urinary incontinence are also at greater risk of persistent genital colonization and relapsing urinary infections.

New Infection or Recurrence of an Old Infection

Most episodes of urinary tract infections are not reinfections. In other words, every UTI is a new infection. This means that each episode of a UTI is associated with a new cycle of contamination and ascending infection of the bladder.

How Does the Bladder Protect Itself From Ascending Bacteria?

The bladder is well protected from the outside by a closed urethra. The closed urethra is the gatekeeper of the bladder that prevents bacteria from entering the bladder. During the time that the bladder fills with urine, the urethra is closed and any crevices are plugged with mucus secreted by the urethra. Bacteria cannot ascend the urethra when the urethra is closed.

During voiding or urination, however, the bladder is vulnerable to ascending infection because the urethra is open. The urine stream is not smooth; it is turbulent. Bacteria that might contaminate the distal or lower end of the urethra can be washed upwards during urination. That is how bacteria enter the bladder: when the door to the bladder (urethra) is open, bacteria can enter. Drinking a lot of water is no protection against urinary tract infection. Drinking a lot of water means lots of trips to the bathroom and more frequent opening of the urethra. The more frequently that the door to the bladder is open, the more frequent the opportunities for bacteria to enter the bladder.

CHAPTER 4:
Ascending Urinary Tract Infections

M OST URINARY TRACT infections are ascending infections, meaning that the *E. coli* that contaminate the urethral area ascend into the bladder through the urethra. Once contamination of the genital area has occurred, it is commonly thought that intercourse pushes the bacterial organisms up through the urethra and into the bladder. This is a very disturbing thought and may not be entirely accurate. Considering how often intercourse takes place at any one time around the world, if intercourse caused cystitis, we would be seeing a pandemic of urinary tract infections.

THERE MUST BE MORE TO ASCENDING INFECTIONS THAN INTERCOURSE!

How Do Bacteria Enter the Bladder?

While the bladder is filling up with urine sent down from the kidneys, the urethra is closed as a way of preserving continence. This closed state prevents urine leakage during the filling phase of the bladder. When the bladder is full of urine, we feel an urge to urinate. When the bladder contracts to expel urine, the urethra opens to allow urine to exit the body.

One might think this flow of urine would flush germs out of the bladder but there is a problem with that line of thinking: there are no germs in the bladder to flush out. Normally, the urine in the urinary tract is sterile. That means there is not a single germ in the urinary tract. However, if germs are hanging around the genital area, for example around the urethra, they may gain entry to the bladder during urination. In other words, bacteria may be flushed *into* the bladder rather than out of the bladder. An open urethra becomes a risk factor for ascending urinary tract infections, but during sex the urethra is closed and the urinary tract is protected from ascending infections (see Figure 8).

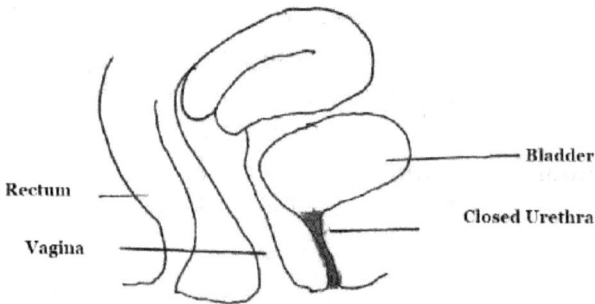

Figure 8: During sex the urethra is closed and the bladder is protected from ascending infections.

How do Organisms Ascend the Urethra During Voiding?

> BACTERIA ARE MOST LIKELY TO ENTER
> THE BLADDER DURING URINATION WHEN
> THE URETHRA IS OPEN. BACTERIA MAY
> BE FLUSHED INTO THE BLADDER RATHER
> THAN OUT OF THE BLADDER.

Dysfunctional Voiding

Dysfunctional voiding refers to interrupted voiding during urination. People who contract the sphincter muscle during voiding and temporarily interrupt the urine stream exhibit a form of dysfunctional voiding. A temporary interruption of the urinary stream may send a squirt of urine from the distal or lower end of the urethra in a backward direction, right into the bladder.

Dysfunctional voiding is very common. Many people routinely contract the sphincter during urination. The habit of contracting the sphincter during or at the end of urination may be voluntary or involuntary. This habit is most often not a problem at all. However, if some *E. coli* find their way to the lower end of the urethra, they can be promptly dispatched upward into the bladder in a drop or two of urine, and possibly cause a urinary tract infection (see Figure 9).

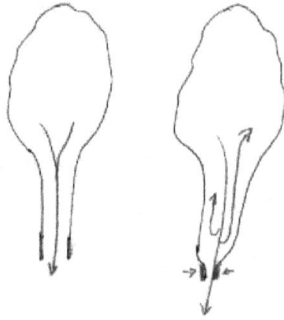

Figure 9: During bladder contraction the sphincter
is relaxed and urine flows smoothly through the urethra.
The second diagram shows dysfunctional voiding:
contraction of the sphincter muscle that causes urine
and bacteria to be washed upwards into the bladder.

The idea that germs, including *E. coli*, enter the bladder during voiding is not a new concept. It is well-known that children who are prone to urinary infections have dysfunctional voiding.

Normal Voiding and Ascending Infection

What if there is no interruption to the urine flow during voiding? The urethra still needs to close at the end of urination, and it is during this normal closure that germs may be gently dispatched in an upward direction toward the bladder.

Urine flows most rapidly in the center of the urethra. Urine along the walls of the urethra may flow very slowly or not at all. At the end of urination, the urethra closes from below upwards. As the urethra is closing, *E. coli* that may have contaminated the lower end of the urethra may be lifted upwards in a drop of urine, through the open urethra and delivered to the bladder. At the end of urination, the urethra once again is shut tight but the bacteria that contaminated the lower end of the urethra have been elevated into the bladder, where they may cause a urinary tract infection (see Figure 10).

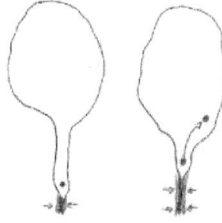

Figure 10: At the end of urination,
as the sphincter is closing,
a drop of urine containing bacteria
can be lifted upwards into the bladder.

Whatever the mechanism, it is likely that bacteria such as *E. coli* have the best chance of ascending into the bladder during urination, when the urethra is open or about to close at the end of urination. An open urethra is a risk factor for recurrent urinary tract infections.

AN OPEN URETHRA IS THE MAIN
RISK FACTOR FOR URINARY
TRACT INFECTIONS.

The urine of those unfortunate people who are incontinent (leak urine) is constantly colonized by bacteria. People who are incontinent have a urethra that is continually open to the environment. They have a steady stream of urine flowing from the bladder through the urethra. Rather than flushing out organisms, the stream of urine permits bacteria from the periurethral area to ascend into the bladder. However, one does not need to be incontinent to be at risk of ascending urinary tract infections.

Frequent urination is a risk factor for urinary tract infection. There is a noted increase in the frequency of urinary tract infections in patients with diabetes and in pregnant women.

Diabetes Mellitus

It is well-known that diabetic patients are at increased risk of developing urinary tract infections. The explanation that is commonly advanced is that diabetics have too much glucose in the urine and glucose favors the growth of bacteria. Another theory is that diabetics have impaired immunity to infections. While both of these explanations may be valid, they do not explain how the bacteria enter the bladder in the first place. The answer is that diabetics urinate very frequently. This means that the urethra opens often which, in turn, increases the number of opportunities for bacteria to ascend to the bladder and cause a urinary infection.

Pregnancy

Urinary tract infections are more common during pregnancy. The usual explanation for the increased risk of urinary tract infections in pregnancy is that the hormones of pregnancy cause stasis or stagnation of urine in the bladder. It is also well-known that there is dilation of the ureter in pregnancy, which may cause a predisposition to kidney infections. However, these changes do not explain why bacteria are more likely to enter the bladder during pregnancy.

The answer is that the enlarging uterus causes pressure on the bladder. Constant pressure on the bladder causes a constant urge to urinate. Frequent urination causes the urethra to open often to release urine which increases the opportunities to expose the bladder to ascending bladder and urinary tract infections.

> FREQUENT URINATION APPEARS
> TO BE A RISK FACTOR FOR
> DEVELOPING RECURRENT
> URINARY TRACT INFECTIONS.

CHAPTER 5:
Urinary Tract Infection Is The Second Most Common Infection

Why are UTIs the Second Most Common Infection?

To UNDERSTAND WHY urinary tract infections are not the most common type of infection, we need to examine respiratory tract infections, which are the most common. Respiratory tract infections include the common cold, influenza, and such conditions as laryngitis, bronchitis, and pneumonia. Upper respiratory tract infections are by far the most common infection to affect mankind. Every year we encounter billions of respiratory tract infections.

Respiratory tract infections are prevalent because the disease-producing organisms are airborne. And since we all have to breathe, all the time, the possibility of inhaling an airborne germ is very likely. Respiratory tract infections are common because the respiratory tract is an open system; it is open to the air at all times. We breathe air through our nose and our mouth about 20,000 times each day. Since either the nose or mouth is always open for breathing, we are constantly at risk of inhaling germs.

The urinary tract is a closed system most of the time. A healthy adult may urinate about six times each day. It is only during urination, when the urethra is open, that the urinary tract is open to the environment.

The urethra is the doorway to the urinary tract so when the door is open, bacteria can enter. When the door is closed, bacteria are barred from entering.

This explains why several billion respiratory tract infections are seen each year compared to several million urinary tract infections. Although urinary tract infections are much less prevalent than respiratory tract infections, they are still the second most common type of infection.

> EACH YEAR SEVERAL MILLION
> URINARY TRACT INFECTIONS ARE
> ENCOUNTERED. URINARY TRACT
> INFECTIONS ARE THE SECOND MOST
> COMMON INFECTION.

CHAPTER 6:
Diagnosis of a UTI

Importance of a Proper Diagnosis

IT IS IMPORTANT to document a urinary infection in a patient who displays UTI symptoms. To document a UTI means proving that the patient indeed has a urinary infection. There are causes of frequent urination and burning upon urination other than a urinary infection.

Documenting a urinary infection is the key to proving that a person has recurrent urinary infections. Some women are convinced they have been having recurrent urinary tract infections when, perhaps, they have actually only had one or two in their lifetime, or even none at all.

Treating a person for a UTI is not proof that they have a urinary infection. To properly manage recurrent UTIs, it is essential that every infection is documented or proven. Many women are labeled as having recurrent urinary tract infections and are treated endlessly with repeated courses of antibiotics. These women receive treatment with little or no proof of the diagnosis. Other women are labeled as having chronic urinary infections and given no hope of a cure, even when actual infections are either rare or nonexistent.

How to Diagnose a UTI

Diagnosing a urinary infection involves laboratory examination. A properly collected urine sample should be submitted for urine analysis and culture.

Proper Collection of a Urine Sample

Urine for a urine analysis and culture is best collected as a clean-catch midstream urine sample. Generally, a lab worker or nurse hands the patient a specimen container and asks her to "pee in the cup."

Women: Once inside the bathroom, open the cup and lay the cap aside in a place that ensures easy access to the open container. Sit far back on the toilet seat. Hold the labia apart to ensure a free flow of urine from the bladder. When a stream is established, insert the specimen cup in the stream until you have collected an inch or two of urine. When an adequate amount of urine has been collected, remove the container from the stream and set it aside. Continue to void into the toilet to completion, with an uninterrupted stream. Stopping and starting is not required during urination. The urine sample is now a midstream, clean catch specimen. Finally, screw the cap firmly onto the container and hand the specimen in for analysis. Make sure the container is well marked ahead of time with your name and identification number. You need *not* wash the genital area prior to collection or wipe the area with an alcohol swab. These precautions do not contribute to the sterility of the urine sample. In fact, they may cause burning and add unnecessary cost.

Men: Once inside the bathroom, begin to void into the toilet. When a stream is established, pass the container into the stream and remove it when an inch or two of urine has entered the container. Continue to void uninterrupted until the bladder is empty. Uncircumcised men should retract the foreskin prior to voiding to prevent contamination of the specimen with organisms that may be present under the foreskin. The foreskin should be restored to its natural forward position following voiding.

After collecting urine samples, both men and women should wash their hands thoroughly with soap and water.

CHAPTER 7:
Treatment of a Bladder Infection

T HE MAINSTAY TREATMENT of urinary infections is antibiotics. Antibiotics are prescribed by a physician or another licensed caregiver.

Antibiotics

A limited array of antibiotics is available for treatment of a UTI:

- fluoroquinolones such as levofloxacin and ciprofloxacin
- tetracycline
- amoxicillin
- cephalosporins such as cephalexin
- nitrofurantoin
- sulfamethoxazole and trimethoprim combination
- trimethoprim alone

Fluoroquinolones are commonly prescribed and are very effective in eradicating urinary infections. They were originally released for the treatment of complex urinary infections. Fluoroquinolones are overused and, as a result, many organisms are now resistant to this class of antibiotics.

Tetracycline antibiotics are used very little these days. Bacterial resistance develops within a day or two, and they are more prone to allow for an overgrowth of yeast in the vagina. Yeast infections are a common complication of antibiotic treatment and often are more bothersome than the original UTI.

Amoxicillin is a type of penicillin that is relatively safe and effective for certain types of urinary infections. *Cephalosporins* are similar to the penicillin-type of antibiotics and are also useful in treating many kinds of urinary infections. *Nitrofurantoin* has proven to be a safe and effective treatment of acute cystitis. The combination drug *sulfamethoxazole* with *trimethoprim* is one of the most commonly prescribed antibiotics for UTIs. There is an increasing resistance of bacteria to this group of antibiotics. Trimethoprim as a single agent is a useful antibiotic that is currently underutilized.

Precautions

People who are allergic to certain antibiotics cannot take those antibiotics. If an allergy develops whilst taking an antibiotic, that course must be stopped immediately, and a physician contacted. Some allergies can be life threatening, such as those that cause breathing difficulty. Severe allergies usually require emergency attention. Only certain antibiotics can be used during pregnancy and only under medical supervision.

Why Certain Antibiotics and Not Others?

Antibiotics are chosen for use in UTIs for two primary reasons: first, they have a spectrum of action that is likely to work for urinary infections; second, they are excreted by the kidneys and therefore develop a high concentration in the urine, which is where the action is required. Since a high concentration of the antibiotic is necessary to eliminate urinary infection, we should not dilute the concentration of the antibiotic in the urine by drinking too much fluid. This would defeat the intention to deliver a knockout dose to the offending bacteria.

Fluids with Antibiotics

All too often, well-meaning nurses or caregivers will instruct people with urinary tract infections to drink a lot of water with their antibiotics. There is a problem with that advice: drinking a lot of water will dilute the concentration of the antibiotic in the urine. This dilution may reduce the effectiveness of the antibiotic and delay the recovery from infection.

Furthermore, watered-down urine will also dilute the natural defenses of the body to fight off the infection. The bladder produces certain chemicals that can neutralize the bacteria and send certain white blood cells to destroy and ingest the bacteria. Too much water in the urine not only dilutes the concentration of the antibiotic, but also thins out the natural defenses of the bladder so they have difficulty finding and eliminating the bacteria.

> TOO MUCH WATER IN THE URINE
> DILUTES THE CONCENTRATION
> OF THE ANTIBIOTIC.

How Much Water Should You Drink with Antibiotics?

The amount of liquid taken with antibiotics should be no more or less than the normal intake required to maintain good health. If a person is inclined to purposely drink a lot of liquid during healthy times, less liquid would be appropriate during an infection. The amount of liquid we drink should be determined primarily by thirst. It is best to use a common-sense approach to drinking, and not drink so little that we become dehydrated and require emergency care.

There are two more reasons to limit fluid intake during antibiotic treatment of a urinary infection. First, in order to realize a cure from antibiotics, every last germ in the urine must be destroyed. Drinking extra fluids may wash out some of the live bacteria, but it is impossible to flush out all of the organisms. Leaving even a few bacteria behind will guarantee failure—as the few will soon become many. Second, drinking extra fluids during an acute infection increases the frequency of painful urination. It is far gentler to reduce the patient's frequency of painful voidings.

Exceptions to Low-Liquid Intake with Antibiotics

There is an exception to drinking less liquid with antibiotics, and it concerns treatment of UTIs with the combination antibiotic sulfamethoxazole with trimethoprim.

Sulfamethoxazole is a sulfonamide type of antibiotic. Sulfonamides have a tendency to precipitate (form particles) in the kidneys and the urinary tract. When that happens, the kidneys may become obstructed by sulfonamide crystals and cause kidney failure. Therefore, patients taking the sulfamethoxazole and trimethoprim combination are correctly advised to increase their fluid intake.

Trimethoprim alone does not have the problem of precipitation in the urinary tract. Trimethoprim as a single agent is a smaller tablet that is a lot easier to swallow. People who are allergic to "sulfa" drugs can still take trimethoprim, which is not a sulfonamide. When taking trimethoprim as a single agent, there is no need to increase fluid intake beyond normal.

Trimethoprim alone is just as effective as the combination of sulfamethoxazole and trimethoprim in eradicating a simple urinary infection. People who develop allergic reactions to the combination of sulfamethoxazole with trimethoprim are more likely to be allergic to the sulfonamide component of the medication. However, since it is impossible to determine whether the person is allergic to the sulfonamide component or the trimethoprim, this combination can no longer be prescribed for future urinary infections. Thus, a person who develops an allergic reaction to the combination drugs may be deprived of using trimethoprim, which could otherwise be a useful agent in treating a future UTI.

How Long Should One Take Antibiotics?

More than half of all UTIs can be cured by a single dose of antibiotics. If the correct antibiotic is selected, nearly all infections can be eradicated by a three-day course of treatment. It is unusual to need more than three days of medication to cure acute cystitis. The exception is nitrofurantoin, which is recommended for five days, but most cases should be cured in three days.

What About Too Many Antibiotics?

All too often, women who complain of burning may be prescribed a longer course of antibiotics, say seven to ten days' worth. However, too many antibiotics can destroy the natural bacteria in the vaginal area. When that happens, a yeast infection may develop in the vagina. The discomfort, itchiness, and vaginal discharge associated with a yeast infection may be more bothersome than a urinary tract infection. This leads to another prescription for the yeast infection and some cream to apply to the area. Also, antibiotics can sometimes cause uncontrollable diarrhea, which may require different antibiotics again.

> TOO MANY ANTIBIOTICS FOR TOO LONG A TIME IS A PROBLEM THAT BOTH PATIENTS AND CAREGIVERS NEED TO BE AWARE OF.

CHAPTER 8:
Self-Diagnosis and Self-Treatment of a UTI

T HERE IS NO good time to get a UTI. An infection can develop suddenly at any time. In fact, UTIs seem to attack at the most inconvenient times. For some unknown reason, UTIs like to strike on Friday afternoons when the doctor's office is closed for the weekend, or on the day you are leaving for a vacation that has been some time in the planning. Women who have had a UTI are familiar with the symptoms and can almost diagnose the condition themselves. If they have a known history of UTIs, they wish to have control when it comes to early treatment of UTIs. They do not want to delay obtaining the prompt relief that antibiotic treatments can provide.

Self-diagnosis and self-treatment of a urinary tract infection is a well-accepted method of managing recurrent acute cystitis. There are several advantages to a self-treatment program. No one knows better than the woman who is experiencing it when a UTI is developing and, most likely, she will not want to wait for an appointment that could delay the start of her treatment. The earlier the antibiotic treatment is instituted, the quicker the infection will be eliminated.

There are several rules to follow when embarking on a self-treatment program. The caregiver should provide the patient with a few sterile urine containers and a supply of antibiotics. At the first signs of a UTI, the woman should provide a midstream sample of urine for urine analysis and culture. At the first opportunity, the specimen should be delivered to the laboratory. If for some reason immediate delivery to the lab is not possible, for example because it is night-time, the sample can be stored in a plastic bag in the refrigerator, not the freezer, for delivery the next morning. In either case, as soon as the midstream urine is collected, the woman can start taking her antibiotics. Thus, early treatment is instituted and a quick response to treatment and a prompt resolution of her symptoms can be expected. Symptoms should lessen in an hour or two. Within 12 hours, symptom relief should be almost complete. If the symptoms persist beyond 12 to 24 hours, the woman should seek medical attention.

The advantage of having given a specimen prior to taking the first dose of antibiotic treatment is twofold:

1. The laboratory can confirm if the patient did indeed have a UTI. This is important information for the patient to know. If the self-diagnosis was incorrect, the correct diagnosis and treatment can be instituted.

2. Within a day or two, the results of the urine culture should be available. If the response to self-treatment is inadequate, the provider will have the results in hand for further management.

It becomes a difficult and frustrating process for the provider and the patient to try to reconstruct a diagnosis a day or two after starting treatment that did not work. Having the results of a urine test taken prior to treatment greatly facilitates ongoing management.

CHAPTER 9:
Risk Factors for a UTI

Diarrhea and UTIs

DIARRHEA IS A common precursor of male and female urinary tract infections. Explosive release of a stool may splatter the toilet bowl and splash contaminated water onto the genital area. Contamination of the periurethral area may lead to an ascending infection of the bladder during the next urination.

A similar sequence of events may occur when preparing for a colonoscopy (an examination of the colon). The bowel preparation to cleanse the colon before a colonoscopy involves ingesting a large amount of liquid that causes watery stool. This poses a threat of backsplash of fecal material, contamination of the genital area and risk of an ascending infection of the bladder.

When passing watery stool, special care should be taken to prevent contamination of the genital area. Floating tissue paper in the toilet bowl can reduce backsplash of fecal material. Of course, the anal area needs meticulous cleaning after each bowel movement, followed by washing the hands with soap and water.

Colostomy Bag

In males, a colostomy bag attached to the front of the abdomen may hang down to the level of the penis. Men who wear a colostomy bag should be careful to avoid contamination of the penis with stool that might leak out of the bag.

Constipation and UTIs

Constipation is common among patients with recurrent urinary tract infections. Difficult passage of stool causes fecal soiling around the anus that is difficult to clean. This results in the potential for genital contamination and ascending UTIs. Regulating bowel movements by moderating liquid intake, increasing dietary roughage, and taking psyllium supplements can go a long way to prevent constipation and UTIs. As always, meticulous cleaning of the anal area is essential to prevent contamination.

Chronic constipation is seen frequently in patients living in nursing homes and long-term care facilities. Immobility and pain medication can lead to severe constipation. Stool above the rectum can undergo fermentation and liquefaction. The watery stools escape around the hard stool in the rectum. This may look like diarrhea, which can lead to a urinary tract infection. Prescribing antidiarrheal agents simply makes the whole situation worse. These patients need an intensive bowel regimen to ensure regularity and the means of getting to a toilet regularly to prevent constipation.

Underwear, Diapers and UTIs

Contaminated underwear presents a risk for transfer of stool bacteria to the periurethral area. Underwear should be checked for fecal stains and changed regularly. Men and women who wear diapers or pads for urinary incontinence or fecal incontinence are prone to develop urinary tract infections. Stool on the diaper may be transferred to the area of the urethra, which can set the stage for ascending urinary infections whenever urine leaks out of the bladder.

Pools and Hot Tubs

It is most unlikely that simply sitting in a hot tub or a whirlpool will cause a urinary tract infection. However, should a person, male or female, urinate whilst sitting in a pool or hot tub, there is risk of developing inflammation of the bladder. During urination, the urethra is open, and water from the pool or hot tub can enter the bladder. If the water contains chemicals, this can cause a chemical inflammation of the bladder. If the water is contaminated by fecal or environmental bacteria, these bacteria can enter the bladder and cause bacterial inflammation of the bladder. Whether the condition is a chemical cystitis or bacterial cystitis, the symptoms are similar. Both conditions will lead to severe pain and burning on urination. Without a urine culture, it would be impossible to distinguish chemical from bacterial inflammation. The best prevention is to not urinate in a hot tub or whirlpool.

If a man should ejaculate inside a hot tub there is an additional risk that contaminated water can enter the ejaculatory ducts and cause severe inflammation of the epididymis. The epididymis, located in the scrotum next to the testicle, stores sperm produced by the testicle. Inflammation of the epididymis is called acute epididymitis. Acute epididymitis causes marked pain and swelling in the scrotum that takes a long time to heal.

Bubble Baths

Bubble baths have been implicated in the causation of bladder infections in children. It seems most unlikely that the bubbles in the bath can go up through the closed urethra and enter the bladder. It is possible that the bubbles in a bubble bath may stimulate a voiding reaction. When a person urinates inside a bubble bath the urethra will open and allow bath water to enter the bladder. Chemicals in the bath water may cause chemical cystitis. If the bath water is contaminated with fecal organisms the result might be a true bacterial cystitis. Both conditions will cause painful urination and a bacterial cystitis will likely need treatment with antibiotics.

TO PREVENT SERIOUS INFLAMMATION
OR INFECTION OF THE BLADDER, A
PERSON SHOULD NOT URINATE WHILE
SITTING IN A TUB, SWIMMING IN A POOL
OR TAKING A SHOWER.

Spermicides

Spermicides are chemicals that kill sperm and are used in an attempt to prevent pregnancy during intercourse. Spermicides are sold as a jelly, cream or foam that the women can insert into the vagina before intercourse and some brands of condoms are coated with a spermicide. The chemical can enter the open urethra when a woman urinates after sex and cause a severe burning sensation. The chemical can enter the male urethra and bladder during ejaculation, and cause alarming burning on urination.

CHAPTER 10:
Prevention of a UTI

IT IS BETTER to prevent a urinary infection than to treat it. However, the ideal of complete prevention is not possible, as contamination and ascending infection is a constant risk. Nevertheless, some effort to reduce the frequency of urinary infections is worthwhile. To understand prevention of urinary tract infections, keep in mind that *UTIs begin in the bathroom, not in the bedroom.* The mainstays of the prevention of UTIs involve hygiene, fluids, diet, urination, and rituals around the time of sex.

THE MAINSTAYS OF THE PREVENTION OF
BLADDER INFECTIONS INVOLVE HYGIENE,
FLUIDS, DIET, URINATION, AND RITUALS
AROUND THE TIME OF SEX.

Hygiene

Cleaning the Genital Area

Only the external or visible genitalia need to be cleaned. During showering or bathing, the external genitalia should be washed gently with soap and water. The area inside the labia has unique protective qualities to keep *E. coli* and other germs at bay. The body's natural defenses prevent unwanted bacteria from inhabiting this area. These defenses help to either shed the organisms lingering in the urethral area or dry them out. Therefore, there is no need to reach inside the genitalia to clean, as the inside is self-cleaning. In fact, washing inside may cause irritation, introduce germs to the periurethral area, and create a risk factor for new infections.

Cleaning the Anal Area

Keeping the perianal (around the anus) area clean of fecal material is most important in preventing future genital contamination and ascending urinary infections.

Showering and Bathing

It is often recommended that women take showers instead of baths. For the most part, that is good advice. But bathing is one of life's natural pleasures, and women with UTIs should not be deprived of taking a hot bath. The risks of taking a bath versus a shower are not great as long as certain precautions are taken.

Many people believe that the rear end is the dirtiest part of the body and, therefore, should be washed first during a shower or bath. But it makes little sense to wash the anal area first because washing the anal area first could encourage fecal material to be spread to other parts of the body. A better idea is to start washing the body from top to toe, then wash the genital area gently. Cleaning the rear end should be left for last. Once the rear end is clean, wash your hands thoroughly.

Before a Bowel Movement

Prior to urination or defecation, it is a good idea to float a layer of tissue in the toilet bowl to prevent an upwards splash of infected material.

After a Bowel Movement

After a bowel movement, dab the genital area with dry tissue, as needed. This should be done before cleansing the anal area. Washing the anal area and the genital area at the same time presents a risk of moving stool to the genital area. Meticulous cleansing of the anal area after a bowel movement is essential to prevent future soiling and contamination. Such cleansing should be limited to the anal area *only*, so as not to contaminate the genital area.

Good hygiene suggests that the anal area first be cleaned with soft dry toilet tissue. When the tissue is visibly clean, the anal area can be further cleaned using several layers of tissue moistened with warm tap water. If available, non-irritating wet wipes are convenient for this purpose. Finally, the anal area should be patted with dry tissue.

Wiping from front to back is common and sound advice to prevent recurrent UTIs. More specifically, all wiping and cleansing should be done with the arms and hands reaching behind the body to access the anal area. Wiping and cleansing of the anal area should not be done by reaching from the front to the back between the legs. To conclude the cleansing process, the hands should be carefully washed with soap and water.

KEEPING THE PERIANAL AREA CLEAN
OF ANY FECAL MATERIAL IS MOST
IMPORTANT IN PREVENTING GENITAL
CONTAMINATION AND ASCENDING
URINARY INFECTION.

Cotton Underwear

Cotton underwear has been recommended for woman with UTIs. Women who prefer cotton should continue to use cotton clothing. Any type of underwear should be free of fecal soiling, which can lead to genital contamination.

Fluid Intake

Perhaps the most common advice given to women with recurrent urinary tract infections is to drink a lot of fluid. Some recommend drinking "a lot" of water, while others specify drinking at least eight to ten glasses per day. If you are following this plan of drinking a lot of liquid and it is working for you, you need read no further. Women who are following an established regimen that works for them should make no changes. However, other women are not as fortunate; they are drinking as much fluid as they can, yet they continue to experience frequent recurrences of UTIs. The commonly-stated goal of drinking a lot of water is to "flush germs out of the bladder" before they can cause an infection. This makes little sense since the urinary tract is normally completely free of bacteria and has no organisms to flush out.

> DRINKING A LOT OF LIQUID LEADS TO FREQUENT URINATION, AND FREQUENT URINATION IS A RISK FACTOR FOR ASCENDING URINARY INFECTIONS.

Drinking a lot of liquid leads to frequent urination, and we have already seen that frequent urination is a risk factor for ascending urinary infections. Frequent urination causes the urethra to open repeatedly to allow urine to exit the bladder. Every time a person urinates, the urethra opens and opening the urethra is like opening the door of the urinary tract and potentially inviting bacteria to ascend to the bladder. This is especially true if there is fecal contamination in the genital area.

While drinking less fluid is not certain to prevent an ascending urinary tract infection, a diet that limits fluid intake may substantially reduce the number of opportunities for ascending bladder infections. Even a modest reduction in the frequency of urinary tract infections is appreciated by those who suffer recurrent acute cystitis.

How Much Liquid to Drink Daily

Each of us should drink as much or as little fluid as we need so as to maintain a normal level of hydration. The amount of water we need can change from day to day. For some, fluid intake depends on their occupation and the weather. People who work in hot environments lose a lot of liquid through sweating and require more fluid replacement while on the job. People who work in temperate climates or do more sedentary work can maintain a normal liquid balance with much less fluid. Nursing mothers need more liquid than non-nursing mothers.

Diabetics may lose so much liquid in their urine that no amount of water can satisfy their thirst. As their diabetes is brought under control though, their intense thirst resolves.

Many people purposely increase their intake of liquid in the belief that water is "good for you" and, therefore, "more is better." This condition is called voluntary *polydipsia*. These people drink more water than their bodies need for normal function and fluid balance.

It is not possible for one person to decide how much water another can or should drink. Natural thirst is the best guide to fluid intake. Some people argue that by the time a person feels thirsty it is too late— that that person is already dehydrated. However, nature has designed the thirst system of the brain in such a way that a minimal amount of dehydration is enough of a trigger to stimulate thirst. Conscious individuals with access to a water source are unlikely to become dehydrated if they respond promptly to the sense of thirst.

Reducing fluid intake may reduce the frequency of urinary tract infections by limiting the number of opportunities for bacteria from fecal matter to ascend into the bladder during urination and, thereby, cause an infection. Furthermore, drinking a lot of fluid will cause some urine to be left behind in the bladder at the end of urination. Urine left behind in the bladder provides a good culture medium for the establishment of a bladder infection.

REDUCING FLUID INTAKE WILL REDUCE THE
FREQUENCY OF URINATION. LESS FREQUENT
URINATION MAY REDUCE THE FREQUENCY OF
BLADDER INFECTIONS.

People with insatiable thirst, such as those with diabetes mellitus, may not be able to reduce their fluid intake. In fact, reducing their fluid intake may place them at serious risk of life-threatening dehydration. The underlying reason for insatiable thirst should always be investigated and treated before any attempt is made to reduce liquid intake.

What if I Have Kidney Stones?

There are five major types of kidney stones. From the rarest to the most common type of kidney stones, they are: cystine, infection stone, calcium phosphate, uric acid and calcium oxalate. Whichever type of stone a patient has, there is a blanket recommendation to drink more water to prevent kidney stones. However, this recommendation is only an adjunct to determining the exact cause of stone formation and prescribing the appropriate preventative or curative medication.

In the case of calcium oxalate stones, which are the most common type of kidney stones, after the tests have ruled out a specific metabolic defect, we are left with the standard advice which is to drink large amounts of water every day. It is well-known that the cause of a calcium oxalate stone in otherwise healthy individuals is dehydration. It is important to understand how and when a calcium oxalate stone forms, in order to effectively prevent a recurrent stone.

When calcium and oxalate molecules join together, they form a salt which is solid. In normal urine, individual calcium and oxalate molecules are held in solution. However, at a time of dehydration, the urine becomes concentrated and there is insufficient water in the urine to keep the molecules in solution. The concentrated urine may become oversaturated with calcium and oxalate. That is when the calcium and oxalate molecules can precipitate to form solid crystals. The crystals of calcium oxalate can quickly latch together to form a kidney stone. This kind of precipitation occurs in the calyces where the kidney joins the collecting system. Once a stone forms, it can grow in the collecting system. At any point in time, sometimes very soon after formation, the stone can drop down into the ureter. A stone in the ureter can block the flow of urine from the kidney and in turn can cause excruciating pain, lower abdominal pain or back pain, on the side of the blockage. The pain of a stone attack will usually send the most stoic of people to an emergency room to get relief.

How Long Does it Take for a Kidney Stone to Develop?

The length of time that it takes to form a kidney stone is much less time than most people would guess. Calcium and oxalate molecules which are normally in solution can precipitate and form solid crystals in a remarkably short space of time, perhaps a few minutes or less. Stones form when a person is dehydrated. Stones are more common in hot climates than temperate climates. It is quite common for a kidney stone to develop soon after a bout of heavy activity or strenuous exercise. It is just at those times that a person may forget to drink extra water.

In temperate climates or when not exerting oneself, fluid intake and urine production is dictated by normal thirst. A problem may arise in hot weather, or at a time of heavy physical activity such as running or cycling, and there is insufficient water intake. During such events, it becomes very important to drink sufficient liquids along the way to prevent dehydration and normal urine production.

It should be clear that in order to prevent calcium oxalate kidney stones, timing is all important. Once a person has become dehydrated and the urine becomes over concentrated, it may to too late to prevent the formation of a kidney stone. A person needs to drink sufficient quantities of liquid along the way to prevent dehydration and the precipitation of a calcium oxalate kidney stone.

Drinking large volumes of water every day when a person is normally hydrated will do nothing to prevent a kidney stone during the next time that a person becomes dehydrated. Drinking large volumes of water every day will simply increase the frequency of urination and thereby increase the risk of a urinary tract infection.

Diet

The purpose of using diet to prevent UTIs is to reduce the frequency of urination and increase the efficiency of bowel movements. We have already seen that reducing liquid intake may help reduce the frequency of urinary infections. But women often ask if other dietary measures are important in lowering the risk of UTIs. The answer is yes, dietary measures can greatly assist in reducing potential contamination of the genital area and resulting ascending infections. Less liquid and more roughage are key.

> DIETARY MEASURES CAN GREATLY ASSIST IN REDUCING POTENTIAL CONTAMINATION OF THE GENITAL AREA AND RESULTING ASCENDING INFECTIONS.

Fiber

The importance of preventing constipation cannot be emphasized enough. The most important dietary measure to consider for bowel regulation is increasing the amount of fiber, also called roughage, in your diet. The goal is to improve the quality of bowel movements, which should be medium soft, easy to pass, and *easy to clean*. A diet rich in fiber is important for bowel regulation. Fiber-rich foods include fruits, nuts, and vegetables—the healthy foods most of us are already aware of. However, most people eat a refined diet that lacks roughage. These people need to supplement fiber by eating whole grain breads and whole grain cereals. Prunes in any form, dried or stewed, are a delicious and inexpensive way to rapidly supplement fiber intake. The whole prune is better than prune juice because the whole prune provides more fiber and less liquid intake. Eating two to three prunes once or twice daily helps regulate bowel movements.

Regular soft bowel movements are easy to clean by wiping the rear end as previously described. Effective cleaning reduces the chance of fecal material contaminating the genital area. Many people question whether increasing water intake can achieve the same result in regulating bowel movements. Unfortunately, there is no roughage in water. Roughage is not absorbed in the intestine; it hangs onto water produced in the large intestine, water which keeps the stool moist and soft. Nearly all of the water we drink is absorbed in the stomach and the upper small intestine. Little if any of the water we drink will ever reach the large intestine; therefore, fluid intake plays no role in keeping the stool soft. Drinking a lot of water may contribute to a brief sense of fullness, but most of the excess water we drink is quickly eliminated by the kidneys and excreted in the urine. At the end of the day, excess liquid contributes little or nothing to bowel regularity but does increase the frequency of urination. And increasing the frequency of urination may be undesirable when it comes to preventing UTIs.

> A DIET THAT IS RICH IN FIBER OR ROUGHAGE, AND LOWER IN LIQUIDS, MAY BE IMPORTANT IN PREVENTING RECURRENT BLADDER INFECTIONS.

Cranberries

There is very little evidence that cranberries can cure a symptomatic bladder infection or that they can prevent an infection in otherwise healthy women.

Urination

When you feel the urge to urinate, do what needs to be done. Delaying urination is not only uncomfortable; it also leads to poor bladder emptying and increased residual urine. These are risk factors that can allow the establishment of urinary tract infections. Prior to urination, it is a good idea to float a sheet of tissue paper in the bowl to prevent backsplash of the potentially infected contents of the toilet bowl. If possible, urination should be a solid stream to completion. Interruption of urine flow may cause bacteria to enter the bladder. Totally avoiding interruption of the stream seems difficult for people to accomplish. Luckily, this is only a problem if bacterial contamination has occurred. The precautions suggested to avoid contamination are more important than the shape of the urinary stream.

The Color of Urine

The natural color of urine is yellow, sometimes dark and sometimes light. In healthy, fully conscious individuals, the color of their urine depends on how much water the kidneys are trying to remove or retain. If the body needs to preserve water, the urine will appear darker, and if the body needs to eliminate extra water, the urine will appear lighter, or even clear. The amount of water the body needs to function normally is finely regulated by the kidneys.

The kidneys rid the body of toxins that build up naturally in the body as a result of metabolism. If the toxins are dissolved in a little water, the urine will appear dark yellow. If the same measure of toxins is diluted in a lot of water, the urine will appear light yellow or clear.

If the body is taking in too much water, the excess must be eliminated to preserve normal body chemistry. In a person who drinks too much fluid, the normal concentration of sodium in sodium chloride, or salt, in the blood stream, can become so diluted that a condition called *hyponatremia*, or low concentration of salt, can develop. A healthy person, even a marathon runner, can develop fatal hyponatremia, by consuming too much water. On the other hand, a person starved of water may become dehydrated. This too is an unhealthy situation and is potentially lethal.

The human brain detects even subtle changes in water balance. If the body craves water, then the brain signals the kidneys to work harder at preserving water balance. The kidneys are obedient and respond appropriately by reabsorbing excess water, which results in darker urine. When a person has ingested more water than the body needs, the kidneys work less hard at preserving water. The kidneys will simply allow the excess filtered water to escape in urine which will then have a lighter color.

CHAPTER 11:
Sex and Bladder Infections

IT IS COMMONLY stated that sex is a risk factor in the causation of bladder infections. The idea that intercourse can force bacteria into the bladder makes little sense. During intercourse the walls of the urethra are apposed and any crevices are sealed by a thin layer of sticky mucus. It is most unlikely that the act of intercourse can massage bacteria upwards into the bladder, along the length of the closed and sealed urethra.

It is well-known that UTIs may occur after sexual intercourse. However, there are many women who experience UTIs at times that are distant from the time of intercourse, or entirely unrelated to intercourse. If sex was the main cause of urinary tract infections, we would likely be experiencing a worldwide pandemic of bladder infections. Clearly this is not happening.

If sex was the primary cause of bladder infections, conventional wisdom would have expected that caregivers advise against sex, to prevent urinary infection. So far, no one has issued such a blanket recommendation. *Instead, a set of rituals were designed around the sex act that were supposed to prevent bladder infections caused by sexual intercourse.*

In terms of preventing UTIs caused by intercourse, the following conventional advice is commonly offered. Women are told to drink a glass of water before sex, wash the anal area and the genital area before sex, urinate before sex, urinate immediately after sex, drink more water after sex, and wash the genital area and anal area again after sex. Not included in the standard recommendations, but often performed by women, is to have a bowel movement before sex.

If a program of drinking water before and after sex, washing the anal and genital areas before and after sex, and urinating immediately after sex is working for a woman, there is no need to change any of these rituals; she should continue as advised.

The problem is that many women, who obsessively adhere to similar rituals, continue to be plagued by recurrent urinary tract infections. Instead of enjoying sex, they may develop an aversion to intercourse, due to a fear of developing a bladder infection. Furthermore, the man who is observing his partner performing all these rituals may develop an unwarranted sense of guilt, that he is somehow part of the problem.

> THERE IS A CONCERN THAT SOME OF THE RITUALS THAT ARE RECOMMENDED AROUND SEX MAY CONTRIBUTE TO, RATHER THAN PREVENT, BLADDER INFECTIONS.

Preventing Bladder Infections Around the Time of Sex

Voiding prior to sex is a very good idea. First, having relations on an empty bladder is more comfortable than doing so with a full bladder. Second, voiding before sex might avert the need to get up immediately afterward to go to the bathroom. Drinking water prior to sex may cause women to get up to urinate soon afterwards because by then the bladder could be full again. If inadvertent contamination occurs during foreplay, then avoiding urination immediately after relations, may protect against ascending infection.

AVOIDING URINATION IMMEDIATELY AFTER RELATIONS MAY PROTECT AGAINST ASCENDING BLADDER INFECTIONS.

A woman who has a bowel movement before sexual relations should pay meticulous attention to cleaning the area around the anus. She need not wash and wipe the inside of the genital area because, as stated earlier, this area is self-cleaning.

Staying in bed immediately after relations has several advantages. First, the woman may wish to remain where she is, to relax. It would seem more natural to stay in bed or fall asleep after engaging in sexual relations. Getting up immediately after relations could send the wrong message to a partner who may feel guilty that he is somehow responsible for causing bladder infections.

Getting up to wash the genital area after intercourse may cause contamination of the area around the urethra. This, combined with drinking water and urinating immediately afterwards, may open a pathway for bacteria to enter the bladder. It is important to allow sufficient time to elapse after intercourse for the body's natural defenses to get rid of any stray organisms that might have inadvertently contaminated the area around the urethra. The tissues around the vagina and the opening of the urethra have properties that prevent *E. coli* from gaining a foothold in the area. Also, drying of the tissues is a potent force in getting rid of unwanted bacteria. It may take a while for the natural defenses and drying of tissues to eliminate potential pathogens from the genital area. If a woman urinates too soon after intercourse, bacteria around the urethra may be flushed upwards into the bladder. This is why it is more prudent to delay urination until the next natural urge to urinate arises.

Vaginal intercourse should not be a cause of urinary infection. However, if a person engages in anal intercourse or anal and then vaginal intercourse, then all bets are off. This type of activity places both partners at risk of urinary tract infections. In such cases, a bladder infection becomes a sexually transmitted disease. Limiting sexual activity to the front end is key to preventing fecal contamination of the periurethral area and ascending urinary tract infections.

CHAPTER 12:
Urinary Tract Infection in Adult Males

Urinary Tract Infection in Infant Males

IN THE FIRST year of life, male infants are twice as likely to develop urinary infection as girls. Uncircumcised boys are ten times more susceptible to infection than those who are circumcised in the neonatal period. Babies with urinary tract infections are usually very sick. They present with a high fever, lack of interest in feeding, and vomiting. It is essential to examine a urine sample for proper diagnosis and prompt treatment of sick babies suspected of having urinary tract infections.

Urinary Tract Infection in Adult Males

Adult men, like women, can develop acute bacterial cystitis. Stool can contaminate the opening of the male urethra at the end of the penis. Bacteria can easily migrate along the penile urethra which is similar to the vestibule of the female. During urination, bacteria may ascend through the membranous and prostatic urethra and enter the bladder. The male can develop acute cystitis, with urgency, frequency and burning on urination. Acute cystitis in males does not produce fever, and responds to a short course of antibiotics, just as in the female.

However, some men may develop a more serious infection due to spread to the prostate. The patient becomes severely ill, with sudden onset of fever and chills, as well as painful, frequent urination. This is a serious infection called *acute bacterial prostatitis*. The patient will usually need to be hospitalized and be given intravenous antibiotics. With the correct combination of antibiotics, the fever will quickly return to normal and the patient will feel much improved. Once the fever subsides, oral antibiotics will be continued for a few more days as prescribed by the treating physician. With the correct antibiotics, the infection will be cured and is unlikely to return, given the proper precautions to prevent contamination in the future.

Prevention of Male UTIs

Hygiene in Males

Hygiene is just as important for men as it is for women. Men should maintain proper cleanliness of the anal area in order to prevent the transfer of stool from the anus to the end of the penis. Men also are advised to wipe the rear end after a bowel movement by reaching behind the body, not by reaching between the legs. Reaching from the front, between the legs, is a recipe for men to acquire a urinary tract infection because on the return forward, after wiping, it is possible for stool to inadvertently deposit on the end of the urethra. If the urethra becomes contaminated, bacteria can enter the bladder during urination.

When bathing or showering, some men feel compelled to wash the rear end first. This is not a good idea, because fecal material may then be inadvertently transferred to the opening of the penis. A safer practice is to wash first from head to toes and wash the rear end last. The hands should then be cleaned thoroughly with soap and water.

Why are Males Less Prone to Contract UTIs?

The traditional reason that is given for this question is that the male urethra is longer than the female urethra. This is not strictly true. The length of the female urethra and the *functional* length of the male urethra are about the same; about four centimeters in both sexes.

In the male, the functional urethra consists of the prostatic urethra and the membranous urethra. The prostatic urethra and the membranous urethra are partly surrounded by smooth muscle which acts as a sphincter to keep the urethra tightly shut. The much longer segment of the male urethra that extends beyond the membranous urethra, traverses the penis. This part of the male urethra is <u>not</u> surrounded by muscle and has no sphincter action.

From a development point of view, the penile urethra is similar to the female vestibule, which is the space between the folds of the labia minora. Bacteria are free to contaminate and move about the penile urethra just as they are able to in the female vestibule.

The reason that males are less prone to develop urinary infections is because the opening of the urethra, at the end of the penis, is further away from the anus and, therefore, much less likely to become contaminated by the stool. However, uncircumcised men may be more prone to urinary tract infections because fecal organisms may settle in the space between the foreskin and the penis.

Chronic Prostatitis

Chronic prostatitis is a common misdiagnosis in men. In the majority of cases chronic prostatitis is not really an infection at all. Men with ongoing complaints related to the pelvic area, such as pain or discomfort in the groin or testicles, are often incorrectly diagnosed as having a prostate infection. These men are usually prescribed repeated, prolonged, and futile courses of antibiotics, and they never really get better. Physical examinations should rule out the presence of other conditions, such as a groin hernia. Active men involved in heavy lifting or sports may develop ligament problems. This can cause pain or discomfort with sitting or heavy lifting. Because these ligaments run alongside the prostate, the prostate may be unfairly blamed for the chronic discomfort. Referral to a physical medicine or sports medicine specialist may be necessary to reach the proper diagnosis and get the appropriate treatment.

It is not uncommon for men to complain of a clear or whitish discharge from the penis during a bowel movement. This is a completely benign condition with a common underlying problem of constipation. As the hard stool leaves the rectum, it massages the prostate and expresses prostatic fluid that appears at the end of the penis. The cure is to prevent constipation.

On occasion, a man may experience severe pain in the ano-rectal area. Once again, the prostate is often unfairly blamed for a pain that occurs some ten to 20 minutes after a bowel movement. In reality, the intense pain is not coming from the prostate but, instead, from a condition called *proctalgia fugax*. This problem expresses itself when a pellet of stool becomes trapped in the anal sphincter after an unsatisfactory bowel movement. The intensity of the discomfort, which can be quite alarming, is due to a spasm of the anal sphincter around the fragment of stool that is caught in place. The condition is immediately cured by returning to the toilet and eliminating the offending piece of stool. Once the portion of stool is eliminated, the pain disappears. To prevent recurrence, constipation must be addressed. Increasing roughage in the diet and taking psyllium every day will ensure complete bowel evacuations. In females, who do not have a prostate, the symptoms of proctalgia fugax may be blamed on the pelvic floor muscles. However, the prevention and cure are the same as for men.

Intermittent testicular pain may be caused by partial intermittent twisting or torsion of a testicle. This condition is rather common in adult men and may be misdiagnosed as chronic prostatitis.

CHAPTER 13:
Preventing Urinary Tract Infection in Females – Review

Why are Females More Prone to Contract UTIs?

THE TRADITIONAL REASON is that the female urethra is shorter than the male urethra. As seen in the previous chapter, this is not strictly true. The functional length of the male urethra and the length of the female urethra are about the same; the main reason why women are more prone to develop UTIs is because of the proximity of the anus to the genital area. It is far more likely for bacteria from stool to colonize in the genital area of women than men.

Another reason is that the traditionally recommended rituals surrounding intercourse may in fact promote rather than prevent bladder infections. Women who experience recurring infections usually urinate immediately after sexual relations, believing that they are 'flushing away' the bacteria in their urethra. However, the urethra is closed during sex and only open upon urination, which is when bacteria will take the opportunity to ascend into the bladder. It is therefore important to empty the bladder before sexual relations, thus eliminating the need to void immediately afterwards, which gives the body time for its natural defences to eliminate bacteria that are lurking in the genital area before the urethra is opened at the next time of urination.

Hygiene in Females

It is crucial for women to maintain proper cleanliness of the genital area, specifically the anal area, in order to prevent the transfer of stool from the anus to the urethra. Meticulous cleaning of the anal area after each bowel movement and floating tissue paper in the toilet bowl prior to urination or defecation can minimize splashback and therefore help prevent bacteria in fecal matter from colonizing in the genital area. Women are advised to wipe the rear end after a bowel movement by reaching behind the body, not by reaching between the legs, so that the chance of stool to reach the urethra is lessened. While genital cleanliness is paramount, obsessive washing of the genital area can predispose women especially to contamination and should be avoided.

When bathing or showering, a top-to-toes approach is best, with the rear end being washed afterward, and the hands washed last. Men and women should not urinate inside a pool, shower or hot tub as it opens the urethra in an environment where unwanted bacteria may be present and can rapidly ascend into the bladder.

Lifestyle

A complete bowel evacuation makes it easier to clean the anal area and reduce fecal contamination of the genital area, therefore it is important to maintain a healthy digestive system. Eating a healthy diet and increasing roughage can ensure regular and complete bowel evacuations that are easy to clean. Many women who suffer from recurrent bladder infections heed traditional advice to drink a lot of water, but moderating fluid intake, thereby reducing the frequency of urination, can potentially reduce the opportunity for an ascending urinary infection.

CHAPTER 14:
Key Messages

A URINARY TRACT INFECTION may develop when bacteria that live in the stool enter the bladder. The bladder is protected from infection when the urethra is closed. Bacteria that cause UTIs enter the bladder during urination when the urethra is open, or at the end of urination as the urethra is closing. We reproduce through the act of interocourse. A tightly closed urethra prevents bacteria from entering the bladder during sex. However, rituals around sex, such as the obsessive washing of the genital area and urinating immediately after sex, may predispose women to urinary tract infections. Prevention of UTIs should concentrate on keeping fecal material away from the genital area. Regular, soft bowel movements and meticulous cleansing of the rear end is most important. Regulating fluid intake reduces the frequency of urination and limits the opportunities for bacteria to enter the bladder.

Following simple measures to reduce the frequency of recurrent UTIs should allow the woman to enjoy a happier sex life and not be intimidated by her bladder.

Glossary of Terms

Acute cystitis: Acute inflammation of the urinary bladder, also called a bladder infection, urinary tract infection, or UTI.

Ascending infection: When bacteria from the outside move up through the urethra and cause an infection in the bladder.

Bladder: The urinary bladder receives urine from the kidneys through both ureters. In its storage phase, the bladder fills up slowly until it contains about eight ounces of urine. When full, the bladder sends a message to the brain that causes a sense of urgency to urinate. During urination, the bladder contracts and expels its contents through the urethra.

Cystitis: Inflammation of the urinary bladder.

Dehydration: A serious condition caused by lack of water. This can be due to starvation and is commonly seen in people who are unconscious. Dehydration can lead to kidney failure, shock, and death.

Escherichia coli: Usually referred to as *E. coli*, these are the most common bacteria to cause urinary tract infections. Other species of bacteria that may cause urinary tract infections include *Klebsiella* and *Enterococci*.

External genitalia of females: Also called the vulva. Includes the clitoris, labia majora, and labia minora.

External genitalia of males: The penis and the scrotum.

Female urethra: A narrow tube about four centimeters long. Urine exits the body through the urethra. The female urethra is embedded in the front wall of the vagina. The upper end of the urethra joins to the bladder at the bladder neck. The mouth or opening of the lower end of the urethra is called the urethral meatus.

Functional female urethra: The full length of the female urethra is almost entirely surrounded by muscle. Therefore the entire urethra is a functional urethra. During the filling and storage phase of the bladder, the urethra and its surrounding muscles act as a sphincter. When it is closed, it keeps urine from leaking out of the bladder. Only during urination does the urethra open up to allow the bladder to expel its contents. At the end of urination, the urethra closes. As a closed system, it is sterile and free of bacteria. When the urethra is open, the urinary tract is open to the environment and prone to entry of bacteria that can potentially cause a urinary tract infection.

Functional male urethra: A tubular structure about four centimeters long. The upper 3 centimeters is surrounded by the prostate gland and is called the prostatic urethra. The lower one cm is called the membranous urethra. Both the prostatic urethra and the membranous urethra are almost completely surrounded by muscle tissue. During the filling and storage phase of the bladder, the functional male urethra is tightly closed and water-tight. During the voiding phase of the bladder, the functional male urethra relaxes and allows the bladder to expel its contents. The urine stream runs through the functional male urethra and along the penile urethra to the outside.

Genitourinary: Relating to the genitals and urinary tracts.

Hydration: Taking in water.

Hyponatremia: A condition in which the sodium level of the body is too low. This occurs when sodium has been diluted by drinking too much water. This is a potentially serious condition that can result in nausea, vomiting, seizures, and death.

Kidneys: A pair of bean-shaped organs located in the back of the abdominal cavity. Their function is to remove the waste products of metabolism and maintain water balance. When there is too much water in the body, the kidneys work less hard and allow the excess water to escape as pale yellow or clear urine. When there is too little water in the body, the kidneys work harder to retain water and maintain water balance. When there is less water in the body, the urine produced by the kidneys appears dark yellow in color.

Labia minora: The so-called inner lips of the external genitalia. Usually, only the lower-most free edge of the labia minora is visible from the outside. Therefore, only the free edge can be said to be part of the external genitalia. The inner aspects of the labia minora are smooth and are in contact with each other. The labia minora enclose a potential space, called the vestibule, into which the vagina and the urethra enter.

Male urethra: Includes the prostatic urethra, the membranous urethra, and the penile urethra.

Male vestibule: Developmentally, the membranous urethra and the penile urethra are analogous to the female vestibule.

Membranous urethra: A short segment of the male urethra that joins the prostatic urethra to the penile urethra. The ejaculatory ducts open on the seminal colliculus in the membranous urethra. The membranous urethra and the penile urethra are equivalent to the female vestibule.

Metabolism: The chemical reactions in the body that enable the body to perform all of its functions. This includes extraction of energy from the food we eat. Metabolism takes place in water, so water is essential for all our metabolic needs.

Over-hydration: A serious condition caused by excess water intake. Voluntary over-hydration, by drinking too much water, can lead to hyponatremia. Too much intravenous fluid given to a patient in a hospital setting may cause weight gain and swelling of the body, and lead to heart or lung failure.

Penile urethra: A tube that joins the male functional urethra to the tip of the penis. The penile urethra has no sphincter function and is not water-tight. The penile urethra conducts urine from the bladder to the outside. The penile urethra is also the conduit for semen at the time of ejaculation.

Penis: Male erectile organ. It contains the penile urethra.

Perianal area: Is the area around the anus.

Periurethral area: The space around the opening of the urethra. The periurethral area includes the vestibule, the opening of the vagina, the opening of the urethra, and the lower one centimeter of the urethra.

Prostate: A male reproductive organ that surrounds the upper three fourths of the functional male urethra. The prostate gland produces about 10-15% percent of the volume of seminal fluid.

Prostatic urethra: The male urethra traverses the prostate. The top of the prostatic urethra runs from the opening of the bladder to the level of the upper border of the membranous urethra which includes the upper border of the colliculus seminalis.

Psyllium: Bulk-forming soluble fiber that comes from the seed of a plant.

Renal pelvis: A funnel-shaped hollow organ that collects urine produced by the kidneys and delivers the urine to the ureter.

Residual urine: The volume of urine that remains behind in the bladder after urination. Normal residual urine should be 0 ml. Even very small amounts of urine may become an ideal culture medium for uropathogenic bacteria.

Ureter: A thin tube that transports urine from the renal pelvis to the bladder.

Urethra: The urethra is a tube that joins the bladder to the outside. During urination, urine flows from the bladder through the urethra to the outside. The female urethra opens in the vestibule. The male functional urethra joins the penile urethra which opens at the end of the penis. See 'functional female urethra' and 'functional male urethra' for more detail.

Urinary tract infection: An infection of the urinary tract, also called UTI, and commonly refers to a bladder infection or acute cystitis.

Urologist: A medical and surgical specialist who treats genital and urologic conditions of men, and urologic conditions of women.

Urology: The study and practice of medicine as it relates to genital and urologic conditions of men, and urologic conditions of women.

Uropathogenic bacteria: Refers to those strains of *E. coli* that are prone to cause urinary tract infections.

UTI: Abbreviation for urinary tract infection.

Vagina: A sheath for sexual relations. The opening of the vagina is immediately behind the opening of the urethra, in the vestibule. In its virginal state, the opening is covered by a membrane with a small opening called the hymen. The cervix or neck of the uterus connects with the upper end of the vagina.

Vestibule: The potential space that lies between the opposing folds of the labia minora. The vagina opens into the posterior section of the vestibule. The female urethra runs within the front wall of the vagina and opens just in front of the vagina into the vestibule. The vestibule is normally listed as part of the external genitals of the female, but rather should be listed as part of the internal genitalia because it is completely concealed by apposition of the labia minora. The vestibule only meets with the outside when the labia minora separate during menstruation and during the delivery of a baby. The vestibule is exposed to the environment when the labia minora separate during sex and briefly during urination.

Vulva: See external genitalia of females.

Water: A tasteless, colorless liquid essential for life and normal body functions, such as metabolism. About 60 to 70 percent of the human body is made up of water. Water is an essential part of our diet. Too little water can lead to dehydration; too much water can lead to over-hydration. How much water we need depends on weather conditions, temperature, sweating, exercise, and activity. We need more water in hot weather and less in cold. When we are active and sweating, our bodies need more water; when we are sedentary, they need less. The amount of water we drink is best determined by our thirst mechanism. The six to eight glasses of water we often hear about include the water contained in our food. Water is essential for life and needs to be consumed in essential quantities.

Water balance: The right amount of water in the body to support normal metabolism. People lose water through the skin by sweating, through the intestines in bowel movements, through evaporation by breathing, and in urine by the kidneys. We take in water through food and liquids. When the body needs more water, our brain tells us we are thirsty. If the body contains too much water, the kidneys produce more urine. The brain and kidneys ensure water balance.

About this Book

D R. POLLEN'S MEDICAL knowledge and experience prompted him to notice groundbreaking patterns and insights into the development and prevention of urinary tract infections. The life-changing lessons in 'Preventing Bladder Infections' will inform the reader of new insights into the causes of recurrent bladder infections and the steps needed to prevent bladder infections. The reader will learn:

- What causes bladder infections
- When bacteria enter the urinary bladder
- How bacteria enter the urinary bladder
- The role of fluid intake and urination in bladder infections
- The roles of hygiene and diet in preventing bladder infections
- Steps to prevent bladder infections during sexual activity

Biography of Author

Jeffrey Pollen MD has studied, practiced and taught urology for more than 40 years. He graduated from the University of the Witwatersrand, Johannesburg, South Africa.

Dr. Pollen joined the University of California, San Diego where he was appointed Assistant Professor in Surgery and Urology. Thereafter he served as a Staff Physician with the Southern California Permanente Medical Group in San Diego.

Dr. Pollen retired after many years of service in the Veterans Administration New Jersey Health Care System.